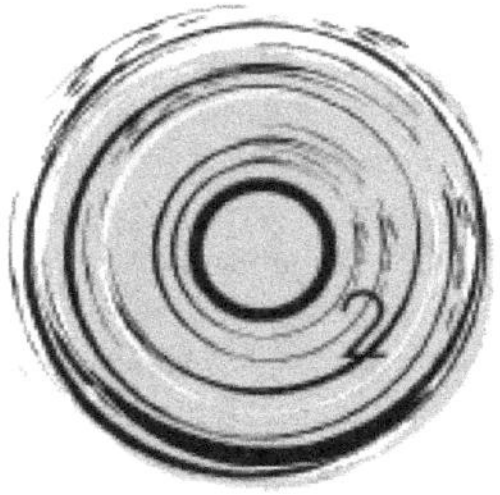

WHY NOT HBOT?

The Battle to Bring Hyperbaric Oxygen Therapy to America's Wounded Warriors

Kevin Hensley

ATTRIBUTIONS
Interior Text Font: Minion Pro
Cover Design & Typesetting: Robbie Grayson III

BOOK PUBLISHER INFORMATION
Traitmarker Media, LLC
www.traitmarkermedia.com
traitmarker@gmail.com

ISBN: 979-8-3495-8427-5

Printed in the United States of America

Table of Contents

Disclaimer

The publisher is providing this book and its contents on an "as is" basis and makes no representations or warranties of any kind with respect to this book or its contents and disclaims all such representations and warranties, including but not limited to warranties of mental healthcare for a particular purpose.

The content of this book is for informational purposes only and is not intended to diagnose, treat, cure, or prevent any mental condition or disease. This book is not intended as a substitute for consultation with a licensed practitioner. Please consult with a physician or healthcare specialist regarding the suggestions and recommendations made in this book.

Traitmarker Media, LLC

A Note
from the Publisher

When I first began publishing, my work naturally gravitated toward the voices of those who served in the War on Terror. These weren't just stories—they were raw combat narratives, firsthand veteran accounts, insights drawn from After Action Reports, and urgent calls for reform within the VA. I believed then, as I do now, that those who have borne the battle deserve to have their experiences recorded with accuracy, dignity, and clarity—and placed where they can influence change.

My sensitivity to these accounts was shaped long before my first book. Born into a military family in 1972, I grew up in Cold War Europe, moving between Department of Defense and private American schools. I saw the Berlin Wall fall, Perestroika crumble, and Communism collapse. These events taught me how decisions made in distant halls of power ripple into the lives of those who serve.

When Kevin Hensley first told me about his idea for *Why Not HBOT?*, I knew it belonged in that tradition. It is the story of the long fight after the war: medical battles, bureaucratic resistance, and a relentless drive to help others still suffering. It is testimony and blueprint: a deeply personal account that becomes a rallying cry for effective care for our nation's wounded warriors, especially those battling the invisible injuries of toxic exposure and brain wounds.

In these pages, you will find both the grit of military service and the grit required to keep fighting once the uniform comes off. I am honored to publish this book—not just as a chronicle of perseverance, but as part of an ongoing mission to ensure that the voices of our veterans are heard, heeded, and never forgotten.

Robbie Grayson | Publisher | *August 2025*

The Purpose of This Book

SINCE 2013, the Veterans Administration (VA) has used the phrase "22 A Day" to describe the average number of veterans who take their own lives each day. Twelve years later—after approximately $3 billion a year and more than $36 billion spent—that number has not gone down.

If you presented a CEO with 22 major problems, were given $3 billion to fix them within a year, and then returned with all 22 problems still unsolved, would you keep your job? Most likely not. The CEO would find someone who could deliver results. Yet here we are in 2025, still accepting "22 A Day" as the norm. In fact, many argue the real number is closer to double. So why is there still no decisive solution for this crisis in the veteran community?

The VA permits certain treatments, but the fight continues to make all viable, non-pharmaceutical options available—especially those that target the root causes of injury rather than just the symptoms. Veterans deserve informed consent, including a clear path to safely taper off medications when appropriate. Too often, mental health care defaults to overprescribed pills, without exhausting every treatment option. Imagine being diagnosed with cancer and told the only "treatment" was to talk about how cancer makes you feel—no chemo, no proton therapy, no radiation. Would that be considered care? That is exactly how too many of our nation's veterans are treated for brain injuries.

That is why we created this Quick Reference Guide on Hyperbaric Oxygen Therapy (HBOT). We believe that when you heal the brain, you heal the body. In these pages, you'll find:

- *My own personal fight for my life and efforts to reform veteran health*

- *Testimonies from veterans, caregivers, and HBOT advocates*

- *Summaries of past, current, and pending state and federal legislation*

- *Research and data supporting HBOT's ability to heal brain wounds*

- *Insight into how HBOT, though currently considered an "off-label" treatment, can be combined with other therapies for even greater results*

HBOT has been shown to reduce suicidal ideation, opioid dependency, incarceration, and divorce rates. The question we seek to answer is simple—yet urgent: *Why not HBOT?*

KEVIN HENSLEY | *August 2025*

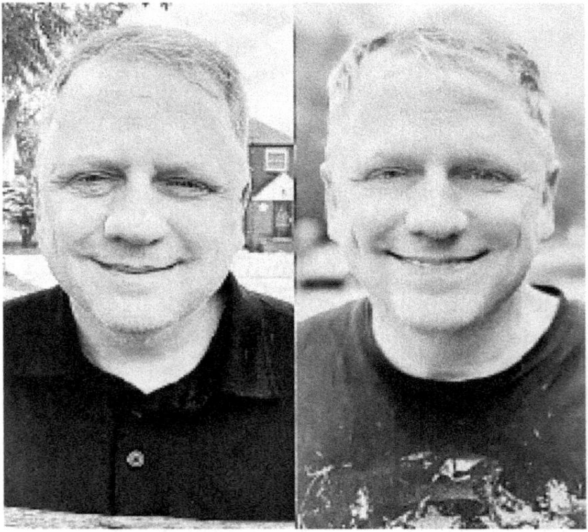

Kevin Hensley
Before & after HBOT
(80 Dives)

My HBOT Story

by Kevin Hensley

I was born in Pontiac, Michigan, in 1975, two months after my family moved to Davisburg. My father worked for General Motors for 28 years, and my parents ran a laundromat for 15 of those, often bringing me along to help. I grew up playing sports with neighborhood friends, attending church every Sunday, and learning the value of hard work.

My family had a long military tradition—my father served in the Navy, my brother in the Army, and cousins in the Navy and Air Force, with an uncle serving in the Marine Corps. By the time I was fourteen, I was working and saving for my first car. High school was a mix of part-time jobs, work-study programs, and occasional trouble with employers over fairness. I met Theresa, who would later become my wife, in French class.

After graduation, I explored my military options, ruled out the Navy after a miserable deep-sea fishing trip, and enlisted in the Air Force in 1995 as a security policeman. Basic training started a week late for me due to a snow delay, which meant I had to catch up constantly. I completed the Security Police Academy at Lackland AFB, trained in law enforcement and security, and became an M60 gunner. My first duty station was Moody AFB, Georgia, where law enforcement and security had already merged into security forces.

Over the next few years, I served in Korea, Jordan, and Saudi Arabia. I patrolled flight lines, guarded gates, and deployed for large-scale exercises. In Jordan, I secured entry points, searched vehicles, and once discovered a man hidden in an engine compartment. My first Middle East deployment was immediately after the Gulf War, where I controlled a no-fly zone and traveled to places like Petra and the Dead Sea.

In the years that followed, I deployed repeatedly: Pakistan in 2003, Iraq in 2006, Iraq again in 2008, Oman in 2010, Kuwait in 2011, and Afghanistan in 2013. I served in roles ranging from patrol to armory management, resource protection, and plans and programs NCOIC. I trained with coalition forces, conducted perimeter security, responded to mortar attacks, and managed security for high-value resources.

It was in Iraq that I first noticed the giant burn pits—open fires consuming everything from trash to vehicles, running 24/7. Smoke and ash would drift over our living areas, coating us as we walked to showers. I inhaled it daily. I got sick—fevers, black and green phlegm—but like most, I was told to "suck it up" and keep working. Over time, I noticed that I couldn't run as I used to. I brushed it off, unwilling to jeopardize my career by reporting health problems that could cost me my weapon and my job.

By 2014, after eight deployments and nearly 20 years of service, I was facing mounting health issues: severe respiratory problems, gastrointestinal polyps, esophageal strictures, chronic pain, and what I would later learn was constrictive bronchiolitis—a terminal lung disease. The VA downplayed my symptoms, attributing them to asthma or COPD despite my never having smoked. It took years, a lung biopsy, and relentless pushing to get the diagnosis acknowledged.

Retirement brought financial strain. Child support consumed most of my pension, our home went into foreclosure, and I struggled with depression and suicidal thoughts. What kept me going was my wife, my children, and the belief that my fight could help others.

In 2020, I connected with Burn Pits 360 and began advocating for legislation addressing toxic exposure. I joined the VFW in Michigan, spoke on podcasts, attended forums, and walked the halls of Congress.

In September 2021, with the help of Burn Pits 360 and their Warrior Hope Network, I traveled to Tucson, Arizona, to begin Hyperbaric Oxygen Therapy (HBOT) at North Star Hyperbaric and Neurology. By the end of October, after completing 80 "dives," my cognitive function had improved tremendously, and my MTBI diagnosis was cleared.

Before treatment, I could barely retain information from a single page. Afterward, I could recall details from books hundreds of pages long. I credit much of this transformation—and the overall improvement in my health and quality of life—to Dr. Henricks and her team.

While in Arizona, I dove into reading about HBOT and its use in brain wound healing. My commitment became clear: once my advocacy work for the PACT Act was complete, I would dedicate myself to pushing for HBOT access for veterans with TBI and PTSD. Since then, I have partnered with several nonprofits and veteran service organizations that support HBOT and are pushing for state and federal legislation—both to treat brain wounds and to expand its use in other areas where research shows significant healing benefits.

Alongside fellow advocates, we pushed for the PACT Act, enduring setbacks, political roadblocks, and personal exhaustion. We staged rallies, confronted lawmakers, and stood watch at the Capitol in the sweltering heat during the "Firewatch" protest.

On August 10, 2022, the PACT Act was signed into law, marking the largest expansion of veterans' healthcare in decades. For me, it meant that if I die within the next several years from my service-connected illness, my family will receive survivor benefits. But it also meant that millions of veterans and their families would no longer bear the burden of proof alone.

I was told one person can't make a difference. They were wrong. My service taught me discipline; my illness taught me the value of urgency. And my advocacy proved that with persistence, teamwork, and truth, we can change the law—and save lives.

Oxygen is the most powerful drug
we never think of as a drug."

Dr. Philip James

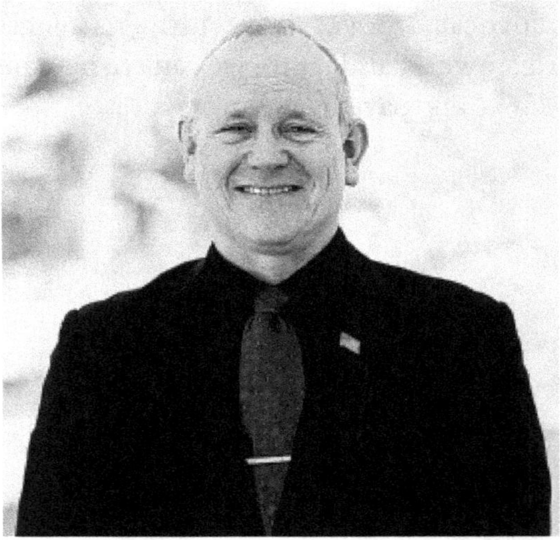

Bob Burton

My HBOT Story

By CSM Bob Burton (Ret)
U.S. Army Special Forces

Restored by HBOT: A Warrior's Journey to Healing and Hope Bob Burton

My name is Bob Burton. I proudly served a 30-year career in the United States Army, retiring as a Command Sergeant Major. Most of my service was within the U.S. Army Special Forces, America's elite Green Berets, where I had the honor of leading and operating alongside some of the most dedicated warriors in defense of our nation.

My career took me around the world in support of national security objectives. I served in the Global War on Terror (GWOT), Operation Enduring Freedom, and I deployed to the CENTCOM

AOR Middle East, including Saudi Arabia, Kuwait, and Iraq; EUCOM Europe, including Germany and France; and across the INDOPACOM Pacific region to countries such as Japan, the Philippines, the Maldives, Thailand, Malaysia, Indonesia, Australia, and Korea. Early in my service, I served in Operation Desert Shield, Operation Desert Storm as part of a multinational coalition to liberate Kuwait, and during Operation Provide Comfort.

Serving in Army Special Operations demanded peak physical and mental performance. The constant operational tempo, training, and deployments stressed my body tremendously. I had years of hard parachute landing falls (PLFs), hundreds of jumps, both static line and Military Freefall, during over 25 years of airborne status. This led to numerous concussions and chronic musculoskeletal injuries, affecting my back, shoulders, knees, and ankles. Like many service members, I pushed through the pain. But after retirement, the cumulative effects became impossible to ignore when life slowed down. My sleep deteriorated, pain intensified, and my ability to function day-to-day diminished. Eventually, I was rated 100% Permanent and Total disabled by the VA due to the physical and neurological toll of my service.

While I can't pinpoint the exact date, the symptoms of traumatic brain injury and PTSD emerged powerfully in the final stretch of my career and worsened during my transition to civilian life. Decades of airborne operations left me with repeated head trauma and concussions that I had minimized at the time. After leaving the military, I began experiencing intense cognitive fog, memory lapses, anxiety, depression, and persistent insomnia. The emotional toll was as debilitating as the physical injuries. I found myself in a dark place, experiencing suicidal ideation, something I never imagined I'd face. Despite all my training and accomplishments, I felt broken. That period marked the lowest point in my life. As a believer, I thank Jesus, that it also became a turning point in my journey to healing.

A fellow veteran invited me to learn more about hyperbaric oxygen therapy. I was skeptical at first, but desperate for relief. I was in constant pain, mentally drained, and emotionally exhausted. After just 10 dives, I started sleeping through the night for the first time in years. My shoulder and back pain decreased significantly. By 20 dives, the physical pain was gone, and my sleep was fully restored. I began to feel like myself again, and I had hope for the first time in a long while.

I completed 40 dives through the HBOT4Heroes program, fully funded by the State of North Carolina. The impact has been transformational. Not only did the pain in my back and shoulders disappear, but the fog lifted from my mind. My PTSD symptoms eased.

Anxiety and depression lessened. At 53, I feel healthier, stronger, and more mentally clear than I did at 43. HBOT didn't just improve my quality of life; it gave me my life back. Today, I'm fully present with my wife and kids, and our relationships are deeper and more meaningful now that I can truly enjoy each moment with them.

It has been over 6 months since my initial round of treatments, and the benefits have endured. That said, I believe HBOT has long-term value, especially for those dealing with chronic conditions or inflammatory issues. I remain open to future treatments as part of an ongoing wellness regimen. It's a therapy I consider a cornerstone in maintaining physical and mental resilience.

To any veteran considering HBOT: Take the leap. This is a natural, powerful therapy that supports healing from the inside out. It reduces inflammation, boosts stem cell activity, and rejuvenates the body and brain. I now serve as an HBOT4Heroes Ambassador, carrying flyers, business cards, and sharing my personal story at every opportunity. I even give out my personal phone number to struggling veterans, because I know what it's like to be in that place, and I know what it's like to come out of it stronger. HBOT was part of my return to purpose and the walk toward fulfilling my God-given potential. I want every veteran to experience the same restoration of hope and health that I have.

If HBOT were a pill,
every VA hospital would stock it.

TreatNOW Coalition

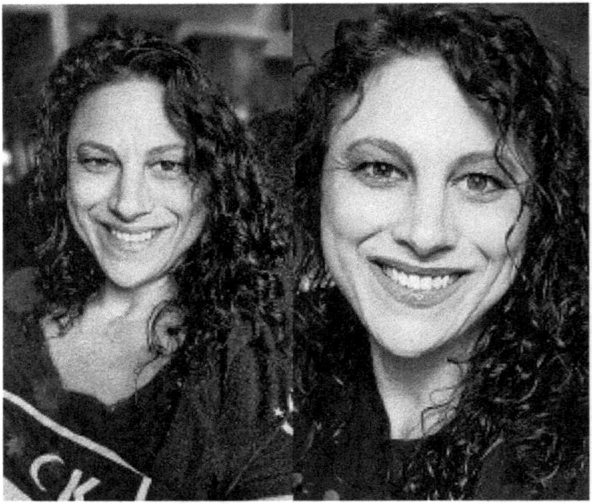

Mindy Dougherty
Before & after HBOT
(Over 25 Dives)

My HBOT Story

by Sgt. Mindy Dougherty USA (Ret)

Before HBOT and Stem Cells: A Personal Testimony of Pain, Healing, and Hope

Before I began hyperbaric oxygen therapy (HBOT) and received stem cell treatments, I was living in a body that was betraying me—collapsing in slow motion while the people around me watched, helpless. Friends could see it in my face, in the way I moved—what little movement I had left.

Once, I could walk the canyon trails with confidence, feeling the earth steady beneath me and the wind brushing my skin. Now, those same trails might as well have been mountains. Every step was a battle my body no longer wanted to fight.

The pain was constant—deep, throbbing, almost sentient, as if it knew exactly when to strike the hardest. My limbs felt like they belonged to someone else, someone whose body was weighted down with cement.

Exhaustion became the air I breathed; I wasn't just tired, I was consumed by fatigue so thick it wrapped around me like a shroud.

My days were sustained by a chemical lifeline—over fifteen pills, each one a bandage on a wound that never closed. The only real break from the pain came from ketamine, which I had to take every other day just to function.

Even that "relief" was blunt, temporary, and carried its own cost. I wasn't living. I was enduring.

When the spiral began, it wasn't just physical. The relentless pain started to erode my mind. My foot would swell any time it hung below eye level, turning a deep, angry reddish-purple that made it look like it didn't belong to me at all. The moment it happened, an electric, burning shock would rocket up my spine and slam into my brain, blotting out everything else.

The inflammation was so severe it began to hijack my thinking, stealing my memory, clouding my focus, warping the way I saw myself. My brain felt like it had short-circuited. I could feel pieces of me slipping away.

Then the darkness came. Not just fatigue. Not just pain. The kind of darkness that whispers you might be better off gone. Suicidal ideation stopped being an abstract concept and became a part of my daily existence. I was scared—not just for my body, but for my mind.

In that desperation, I reached out to Robbie Grayson. I asked if he could help me get sponsored for a home HBOT system. I needed something—anything—to stabilize me before I could even attempt the stem cell therapy my doctors recommended. I knew without it, I might not make it to that next step.

When I finally began HBOT, I had no idea just how profound the change would be. Over the course of 25+ treatments, my body began to remember itself. The swelling in my foot began to lessen. The angry purple faded to the natural color of living skin.

For the first time in what felt like forever, I could place my feet flat on the ground without flinching, without bracing for a lightning strike of pain.

And then came the stem cell therapy—possible only because HBOT had first stabilized me. Together, these two treatments turned the tide. The burning sensations that once defined my days diminished to a faint hum.

Circulation returned to my limbs, oxygen flooded my cells, and the tissue damage that had threatened amputation began to heal.

My brain, once fogged and fractured, started to clear. My memory sharpened. I could think again. I could be again.

HBOT gave me more than relief—it gave me a future. Today, I have a home HBOT system, and it is nothing short of a lifeline. It is the reason I can walk across a room without fear, the reason I can plan days and weeks ahead instead of surviving hour by hour.

For those battling chronic, debilitating conditions—especially those rooted in inflammation, trauma, or poor oxygenation—HBOT is not a luxury. It is not "alternative medicine." It is essential.

Whether your struggle is from burn pit exposure, pulmonary disease, diabetic neuropathy, PTSD, insomnia, surgical wounds, or the suffocating weight of suicidal thoughts, HBOT offers something rare: a non-invasive, life-saving intervention that can restore not only your health, but your hope.

If you are reading this and wondering whether it's worth trying—whether it's worth fighting for—let my story be your answer. It is worth it. It might just save your life, the way it saved mine.

HBOT creates a paradox: flooding the body with oxygen tricks it into thinking it's starved for air—kickstarting repair and regeneration."

Dr. Michael Ruscio, DC

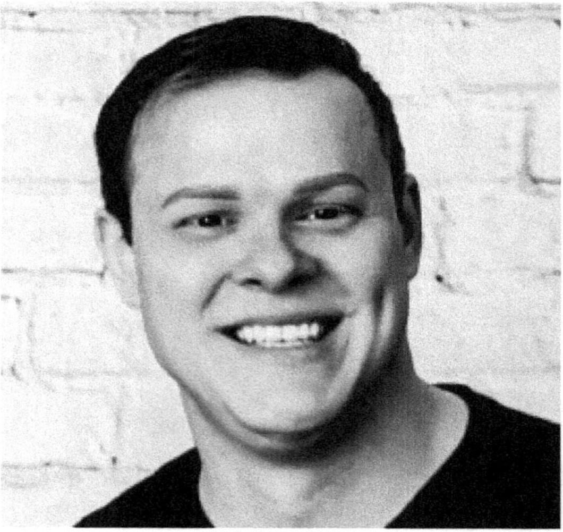

Blake Richardson

My HBOT Story

by Blake Richardson, Sgt (E-5), USMC

Before HBOT and Stem Cells: A Personal Testimony of Pain, Healing, and Hope

While on my first deployment in Iraq (2005), we went through a period when we received indirect fire a few times a week. While sleeping in a general-purpose (GP) tent, a rocket-propelled grenade (RPG) hit the sandbags right outside the tent. After the blast, a Sergeant came into the tent yelling my name, shaking me, and telling me to get up, put my flak jacket and Kevlar on, and get into the bunker. It wasn't until I stood up and started gearing up that I realized I was dazed and had urinated on myself.

The second injury happened while in garrison during helicopter crash survival training. While going through the training blindfolded, I let go of the seat while underwater and upside down. When I tried to get out, I was pushing on the seat instead of the window. Thinking I was free, I attempted to swim out but was still trapped in the simulator. I started to panic and inhaled water until I began to black out and everything became eerily peaceful. A scuba diver noticed and pulled me to the surface, where I coughed up all the pool water.

When did you receive a diagnosis of TBI and/or PTSD, or both?

I was diagnosed with PTSD in 2009. My TBI was identified much later, in 2019, after going undiagnosed for years.

In 2021, a combat-wounded Army Ranger amputee reached out to Help Our Heroes asking for financial assistance for lodging, food, and other costs while going through an HBOT retreat at the Hyperbaric Health and Wellness Foundation in Hailey, Idaho. This veteran was severely struggling with PTSD and TBI symptoms, and his marriage was on the verge of collapse. After completing 40 HBOT dives, he was a completely different person. Not only were his symptoms significantly improved, but he was also able to walk without his cane—and he had hope again. Seeing that transformation drove me to look deeper into HBOT treatment. I eventually connected with TreatNOW, who referred me to the Hyperbaric Healing Institute in Kansas City, Missouri.

To date, I have completed 43 dives. I can now fall asleep and stay asleep through the night. I no longer isolate myself from my family. I am more active and take better care of myself physically. I can read a book and actually remember what I read. My depression and anxiety have drastically improved. I can more easily recall and talk about traumatic events in detail. I now try to get out and spend more time with family and friends. I am more motivated and positive about life. My migraines and headaches have significantly decreased. I can more easily recall conversations and concentrate on tasks. I am less irritable, and I no longer have anger outbursts or mood swings like I did before. I have more energy, I am more organized—and most importantly, I actually have hope.

It has been about a year since I completed my first round of 40 treatments, and I am now getting additional HBOT sessions. I have been told I may need closer to 60 dives to achieve the level of healing I need to regain more normalcy.

I help other Veterans and first responders struggling with PTSD and TBI through Help Our Heroes by connecting them to HBOT facilities that treat at no cost or at a reduced price. I always ask everyone interested in HBOT, "What is your mental health worth to you?" HBOT is a short-term commitment with long-term, life-changing effects. Lastly, I always encourage people to complete the full series of treatments and not to give up.

HBOT doesn't just treat symptoms—
it helps the brain repair itself.

Dr. Shai Efrati

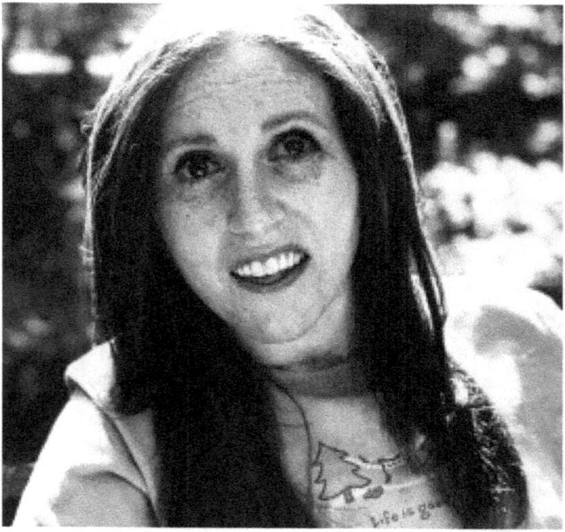

KIMBERLY FIX

My HBOT Story

by Karee White

(*Kimmy's military caregiver & mother*)

about Capt Kimberly Fix, USA (Ret)

Nothing Good Happens after Midnight

They say nothing good happens after midnight. At 2 a.m., the phone rang. Kimmy was on life support at San Bortolo Hospital in Vicenza, Italy.

She had survived a year-long deployment at Forward Operating Base Shank, one of the most dangerous outposts in Afghanistan's eastern corridor. Her job placed her right in the path of constant IED threats where troops and supplies funneled through that base, and every day brought new risk. She came home with PTSD, but she was managing. She had reintegrated at her duty station in Italy and was back to being dependable Kimmy. She was a solid, mission-focused leader who got the job done.

That night, she was the designated driver, doing the right thing, getting one of her soldiers home after a unit "hail and farewell." Somewhere on the Italian highway, a group of teenagers hit her from behind. The impact spun her vehicle, and a second car hit her head-on. She was wearing her seatbelt, but it didn't matter. The forces at play were unforgiving. The trauma to her brain was massive. She suffered a diffuse axonal injury. It's the kind of brain injury where connections in the brain stretch and tear microscopically, often beyond repair.

My husband and I were on a plane within 24 hours. We stood by her side through the medevacs, first to Landstuhl, then to Walter Reed. She never woke up. She was intubated, unresponsive, and officially in a coma. Her Glasgow Coma Scale score was 3 out of 15, the lowest score possible without being declared brain dead. And still, somehow, she survived.

Her body "stormed" constantly. There were episodes where her temperature would spike on one side and drop on the other, her nervous system misfiring uncontrollably. There were so many moments when we thought, "This is it." But each time, Kimmy fought her way back.

After more than a year in a coma, the doctors finally classified her as "minimally conscious." But the vibrant, smart, redheaded Army captain was gone. In her place was a fragile, silent figure who needed 24/7 care. The brain injury had rippled through every part of her body. Her endocrine system failed, and by 29 she had entered menopause. She lost bone density and broke bones easily. She developed drop foot from the months in bed. We eventually had to release the tendons in her legs. We were told over and over that she would never walk, never speak, never progress.

But we brought her home.

We made it work. For ten years, we did everything possible to keep her out of a nursing home. She was in and out of the ICU, at least one hospital emergency every year. Her respiratory system was compromised, and seizures hovered constantly on the edge of our lives. But still, we kept going.

Then I heard about Hyperbaric Oxygen Therapy (HBOT) and a nonprofit called HBOT4Heroes.

Veterans like me were talking about its benefits for brain injuries, and I got connected with Jim Hooker. He encouraged me to give it a try with Kimmy. I was skeptical, but he was persistent and hopeful. Then I met Edward Di Geronimo, who didn't flinch when I described how severe Kimmy's injuries were. Instead, he said, "She'll need every bit of 200 dives."

So we did.

Every single HBOT session, or "dive", involves sitting in a pressurized chamber where the patient breathes 100% oxygen. The science says it helps reduce inflammation, create new blood vessels, and encourage healing even in long-damaged tissue. I didn't know if it would work. But I went into every dive with her. I held her hand, talked her through the transitions, and watched closely.

After just a few weeks, something started to shift.

Her eyes became brighter. She was more alert, more responsive. Her muscle tone improved. Her limbs moved with purpose. She smiled more. She started reaching out with intention, tracking us with her gaze, reacting faster. Her strength returned, not just physically, but in presence. She felt more "there."

Now, we've completed nearly 180 dives. She's stronger than I've seen her in years. A few years ago, she fell and broke her femur. Today, she could beat me in an arm wrestle. Her body is no longer brittle. I don't hold my breath anymore every time she's transferred or moved. We've stabilized. Her health isn't something I panic about every second. And even though she's still nonverbal, she's quick. She's vibrant. She's alive.

HBOT didn't just improve her; it changed what we thought was possible. What I thought was gone in her isn't gone.

We're not chasing miracles. We're building on progress. We've shifted from simply preserving her life to expanding it. We're exploring new therapies, more movement, more hope. HBOT gave Kimmy back a quality of life that the brain injury had stolen. It's given me the ability to breathe again, to stop waiting for the next crisis, and start looking forward.

Kimmy's brain injury was labeled "catastrophic." And it was. But she's proving that healing doesn't end at the one-year

mark. Or five. Or ten.
With every dive, she's still healing.

A 90-day oxygen therapy regimen gave me the biology of a 10-year-old.

Bryan Johnson
(Biohacker)

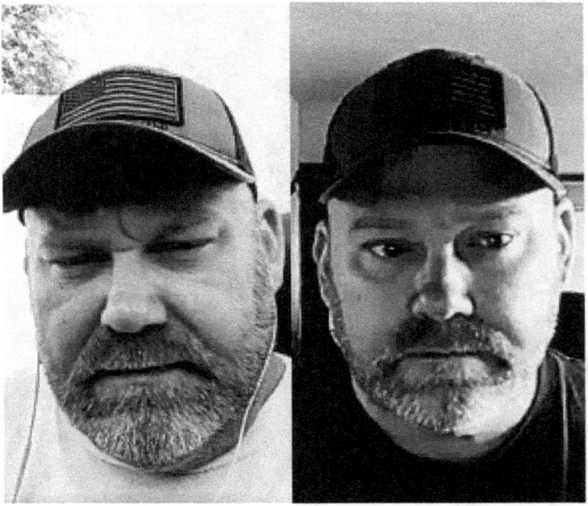

William Wisner
Before & after HBOT
(100 Dives)

My HBOT Story

BY SSG WILLIAM WISNER (E-6)
U.S. ARMY

Deployed to Iraq (OIF V)
from March 2007 to June 2008

I SUSTAINED MULTIPLE concussions from blast-related incidents, including IEDs, rockets, and kinetic entries during raids. I also endured numerous toxic exposures—heavy metals, living in the Al-Tuwaitha nuclear complex in Iraq, COP Casche, and burn pits. While serving as a Bradley gunner in South Korea, we removed the exhaust bags from the auto-cannon inside the turret for expediency during Area 1 operations. Over two gunnery rotations, I fired many rounds, breathing in the exhaust.

I was diagnosed with both TBI and PTSD. My cognition was seriously impacted and progressively worsening. I made contact with Dr. Carol Henricks, a neurologist in Tucson, Arizona, who was working with NFL players for CTE and was also interested in veterans with TBI and toxic exposures.

I completed 110 dives at 1.5 ATA or better. My cognition greatly improved, and prior surgical sites on my Achilles tendons in both legs were positively affected. Before HBOT, I lacked full range of motion in my feet and needed a cane to walk—HBOT restored my mobility. The VA also botched a cancer surgery on my left arm, slicing through lymphatic ducts and leaving me with lymphedema. HBOT significantly reduces the painful swelling that comes with it.

It has been four years since my HBOT treatment. I'm still physically in better shape regarding the surgical site impacts and largely in terms of cognition. However, I remain very toxic from heavy metals, which continue to affect me. I now maintain a 1.3 ATA home bag chamber and an IR sauna, which help with ongoing maintenance.

HBOT was nothing short of life-changing for me. Housing during the process was the most difficult part. I rented a house in Tucson for three months while completing over 100 dives. My doctor wanted to double the protocol because I had so many issues, and I believe that was the right call—I saw incredible gains between 60 and 100 dives. The 1.5 ATA or greater pressure is critical. Bag chambers are excellent for maintenance and far better than nothing, but steel tanks are the ideal starting point.

Hyperbaric oxygen therapy ... is an amazingly simple treatment with huge results.

WASHINGTON HYPERBARIC
OXYGEN THERAPY CENTER

RES
OUR
CES

Core Nonprofits & Clinics

***

Quick tips

Funding/eligibility varies by state and program. Call first to verify coverage or scholarships. If a veteran is in crisis, contact the Veterans Crisis Line ***(Dial 988 then press 1),*** *then follow up with one of the HBOT resources that follow:*

HBOT 4 HEROES

(NORTH CAROLINA)

(919) 874-5754
support@hbot4heroes.org
2012A TW Alexander Drive, PO Box
13887, Durham, NC 27703

Rocky Mountain Hyperbaric Association for Brain Injuries

(Colorado)

(303) 442-4124
jesus@rockymountainhbot.com
225 W South Boulder Rd, Suite 101,
Louisville, CO 80027

NorthStar Hyperbaric

(Arizona)

(520) 229-1238 & 520-229-2122
info@northstarhbot.com
7598 N La Cholla Blvd,
Tucson, AZ 85741

Healing Arizona Veterans

(Arizona)

(520) 222-6036
healingazvets@gmail.com
P.O. Box 64242
Tucson, AZ 85728

Harch Hyperbaric Therapy (LA)

(504) 309-4948
hbot@hbot.com
3409 Division St., Suite 201,
Metairie, LA 70002

TREATNOW COALITION

(national network/help desk)

(571) 549-4268
3816 18th Street North,
Arlington, VA 22207

TreatNOW YouTube channel

(stories, explainers)

Help Our Heroes National

(assists vets & families)

Community Foundation of NC East – HBOT for Vets

(NC program gateway)

(252) 756-8549

Grunt Style Foundation

(national nonprofit; veteran support, HBOT storytelling & advocacy)

Michigan Commanders Group

(coalition of veteran service orgs—policy & referrals)

USF Health HBOT Clinical Trial (FL)

(recruiting veterans & service members)

(813) 396-9200

Cape Fear Living

International Hyperbarics Association

International Board of Undersea Medicine

ANDI INTERNATIONAL

National Board of Diving & Hyperbaric Medical Technology

American College of Hyperbaric Medicine

WARRIOR HOPE NETWORK
BURNPITS360

HBOT
Veteran Links

***

American Grit

(memorial day)

End Dependence Day

Suicide Prevention

HBOT and PTSD

USMC Coalition

VHA Withholding

HBOT News

(special report)

Hyperbaric Oxygen Therapy Helps Veterans Suffering from PTSD & TBI

(parts 1–2)

Helping PTSD Patients Using Hyperbaric Oxygen

NC Veterans with PTSD

(brain trauma eligible for free HBOT)

Dr. Harry van Loveren: Leading TBI & HBOT

(research for veterans —
USF Health feature)

TreatNOW
(channel & curated veteran videos)

Dan Campbell
(Vietnam veteran story)

A Veteran's healing of TBI & PTSD with HBOT

(Bobby Dawson)

Military veteran uses HBOT for combat-related TBI

(interview format)

MAKING HBOT ACCESSIBLE FOR VETERANS

(with veteran Kevin Hensley)

TOC Talks archive

(episodes featuring HBOT clinicians & cases)

Memorial Day 2024

(lest we forget)

Key Studies on Veterans & HBOT

***

Case Series of 39 U.S. Veterans with Mild TBI

(treated with HBOT)

HBOT Improves Symptoms, Brain Micro-structure & Functionality

(in Veterans with Treatment-Resistant PTSD)

Use of Hyperbaric Oxygen for Veterans with PTSD

Broad Mechanistic Reviews

***

HBOT for TBI

(VA evidence brief, 2025)

HBOT for Traumatic Brain Injury

Medical Gas Research

ScienceDirect Overview

Mechanism & Prevention of HBOT-Induced Convulsions

Mechanisms in TBI

The use of hyperbaric oxygen for veterans with PTSD

Hyperbaric oxygen therapy improves symptoms

Hyperbaric medicine

Hyperbaric oxygen therapy compared to pharmacological intervention

Identifying the Target Traumatic Brain Injury Population

U.S. Department of Veterans Affairs (VA)

Veterans & Community Resources

***

HBOT FOR VETS

(NC EAST)

VETERANS IN PAIN (VIP)

Help Our Heroes

Veterans of Foreign Wars (VFW)

USF HBOT
Clinical Trial

International Articles & Testimonials

***

Israeli Soldiers Treated for PTSD

Israeli Breakthrough in PTSD Treatment

Pro Athletes Who Use HBOT

Hyperbaric Medicine International

Hyperbaric Chamber & Sleep

Hyperbaric Nursing PDF

European HBOT (services & technology)

HBOT Pricing Guide

Rocky Mountain Hyperbaric Association

Why Combat Veterans are Turning to Oxygen Therapy

HBOT
Legislation & State by State

***

2014 – OKLAHOMA

Oklahoma Veterans Traumatic Brain Injury Treatment and Recovery Act (SB 1604)

Enacted April 30, 2014, the first state in the nation to pass HBOT legislation for veterans. Legislation in 2023/2024 is in preparation to appropriate funds into a State Fund for treatments. Patriot Clinics have already treated 600+ veterans, first responders, and National Guard members through donations and pro bono work.

Stats: 266,513 veterans; 280 homeless; 13,156 TBI/PTSD; 110 suicides/year; 1,020 with opioid use disorder.

Votes: House 83–0, Senate 43–0

2017 – INDIANA

Indiana Veteran Recovery Pilot Study
(Senate Enrolled Act No. 96 / HB 1306)

Enacted and effective July 1, 2017. Created a five-year, \$1M state-funded program for HBOT, later extended multiple times.

Stats: 380,000 veterans (32,000 women); 572 homeless; 18,210 TBI/PTSD; 153 suicides/year; 1,428 with opioid use disorder.

Votes: House 92–0, Senate 45–0

2017 – Texas

Veterans Recovery Pilot Program (HB 271)

Enacted May 29, 2017; effective September 1, 2017. Provided HBOT via donated/pro bono services from four clinics. Legislation underway to appropriate state funds.

Stats: Second-largest veteran population in U.S.; 1,806 homeless veterans; 68,326 TBI/PTSD; 569 suicides/year; 5,304 with opioid use disorder.

Votes: House 139–0, Senate 29–1

2018 – Arizona

Hyperbaric Oxygen Therapy for Military Veterans Fund (HB 2513 / 1512, Section 26-105)

Enacted March 29, 2018. Appropriated \$25,000 from General Fund for FY 2018–2019 to fund HBOT for military veterans.

Stats: 496,000 veterans; 910 homeless; 22,253 TBI/PTSD; 183 suicides/year; 1,700 with opioid use disorder.

Votes: House 59–0, Senate 30–0

2018 – Kentucky

Colonel Ronald D. Ray Traumatic Brain Injury and Treatment Act (HB 64, KRS 217.930-942) & House Concurrent Resolution 40

HB 64 enacted July 14, 2018 (no state funding); HCR 40 enacted March 30, 2022 urged VA inclusion in HBOT pilot programs. KY Veterans Program Trust Fund provided \$8,000 in 2021 for HBOT.

Stats: 267,000 veterans; 447 homeless; 12,872 TBI/PTSD; \$484.2M annual societal cost; 110 suicides/year; 1,020 with opioid use disorder.

Votes: HB 64 – House 89–0, Senate 38–0; HCR 40 – House 97–0, Senate 38–0

2019 – North Carolina

House Bill 50 / SL 2019-175 (S149)

Enacted July 26, 2019. Authorized HBOT prescriptions for veterans with TBI/PTSD; \$250,000 allocated. Private funding continues to support treatments.

Stats: 667,035 veterans; 31,161 TBI/PTSD; 907 homeless; 256 suicides/year; 2,380 with opioid use disorder.

Votes: House 112–0, Senate 42–0

2019 – Florida

Alternative Treatment Options for Veterans (CS/CS/HB 501)

Enacted June 26, 2019; effective July 1, 2019. HBOT included among five alternative treatments for veterans. Initial \$200K funding, increased to \$14M in 2023.

Stats: 1,525,400 veterans; 67,936 TBI/PTSD; 2,472 homeless; \$3.8B annual societal cost; 562 suicides/year; 5,236 with opioid use disorder.

Votes: House 114–0, Senate 40–0

2021 – Wyoming

House Joint Resolution HJ 0001 – Traumatic Brain Injury and Post Traumatic Stress Treatments

Enacted February 9, 2021. Urges U.S. Congress to enact legislation granting veterans access to HBOT.

Stats: 2,032 TBI/PTSD veterans; 15 suicides/year; 136 with opioid use disorder.

Votes: House 57–3, Senate 4–0

2022 – Maryland

Title: The David Perez Military Heroes Act (SB 709)

Enacted May 29, 2022. Creates a \$1M non-lapsing fund for HBOT treatment of TBI/PTSD veterans.

Stats: 17,409 TBI/PTSD veterans; \$584.5M annual societal cost; 146 suicides/year; 1,360 with opioid use disorder.

Votes: House 135–0, Senate 46–0

2023 – Virginia

Virginia Veteran TBI and PTSD Treatment and Recovery Act (SB 1082)

Enacted March 26, 2023. Allows the Department of Veterans Services to contract with HBOT clinics or accredited hospitals for TBI/PTSD veterans certified by the VA.

Stats: 30,958 TBI/PTSD veterans; \$2.1B annual societal cost; 256 suicides/year; 2,380 with opioid use disorder.

Votes: House 96–0, Senate 36–0

2025 – MISSOURI

Missouri HBOT Veterans Study Bill

Enacted July 2025. Directs a state-led study on HBOT for veterans with TBI/PTSD to assess feasibility, cost, and outcomes for potential statewide adoption.

Books

***

Foundational & Clinical Textbooks

Textbook of Hyperbaric Medicine (6th ed.) by K.K. Jain | A definitive clinical reference detailing history, physiology, equipment, safety, clinical applications, and global practices in HBOT.

Hyperbaric Oxygen Therapy: Principles and Applications by M. Gupta & I. Somasundaram (2024) | Explains mechanisms of HBOT, indications, contraindications, safety, and emerging uses like aging and regenerative therapy.

Physiology and Medicine of Hyperbaric Oxygen Therapy by Neuman & Thom (2008) | A thorough exposition of the physiology, gas laws, and clinical implications of HBOT—critical for practitioners.

Veteran & Rehabilitation-Oriented Reads

The Oxygen Cure: A Complete Guide to Hyperbaric Oxygen Therapy by William S. Maxfield (2017) | Accessible guide with case histories, including on TBI and PTSD treated in veterans, emphasizing HBOT's cellular and holistic benefits.

PTSD and Traumatic Brain Injury Among Servicemembers: Reviews of Medication Practices and Research on Hyperbaric Oxygen Therapy, edited by Tanya Rivera (2025) | A collection of reviews focused on HBOT's role in managing TBI and PTSD in service members, paired with other pharmacological insights.

Specialty & Operational Resources

The Art and Science of Hyperbaric Medicine by Joe Dituri & Jason Sonners (2024) | Modern, practice-focused textbook exploring both standard and off-label uses, mechanisms, safety, and regulatory frameworks.

Hyperbaric Medicine Practice (5th ed.), edited by Dr. Harry T. Whelan | A comprehensive two-volume reference covering the full spectrum of undersea and hyperbaric medicine with contributions from 70 global experts.

Hyperbaric Facility Safety: A Practical Guide | A concise, authoritative resource designed to help healthcare professionals, technicians, and administrators ensure safe operations in hyperbaric environments.

Hyperbaric Medicine Indications Manual (15th ed.) | The definitive guide to the approved uses of hyperbaric oxygen therapy, published by the Undersea and Hyperbaric Medical Society (UHMS).

History & Foundational Literature

Underwater Medicine and Related Sciences: A Guide to the Literature is edited by Charles W. Shilling & Margaret Werts. Annotated bibliography and literature index foundational in both diving and hyperbaric medicine.

Bennett & Elliott's Physiology and Medicine of Diving (Saunders Ltd.) | A classic work exploring diving physiology and HBOT's undersea origins. Includes contributions from Simon Mitchell.

Beyond Normal by Dr. Shai Efrati (2024) | Though broader in scope, this book introduces "enhanced medicine" concepts grounded in HBOT research and its impact on brain healing and resilience.

The Use of Hyperbaric Oxygen for Veterans with PTSD | Explores the emerging application of hyperbaric oxygen therapy (HBOT) as a potential treatment for post-traumatic stress disorder in military veterans.

Textbook of Hyperbaric Medicine | A foundational reference that offers an in-depth exploration of the science, clinical applications, and therapeutic principles of hyperbaric oxygen therapy.

Hyperbaric Oxygen Therapy: Principles and Applications | Provides a comprehensive overview of the science, mechanisms, and clinical use of hyperbaric oxygen therapy. (HBOT).

Physiology and Medicine of Hyperbaric Oxygen is a comprehensive academic text that delves into the biological mechanisms and clinical applications of hyperbaric oxygen therapy (HBOT).

The Oxygen Cure by Dr. William S. Maxfield | Presents a compelling case for hyperbaric oxygen therapy (HBOT) as a transformative treatment for a wide range of medical conditions.

PTSD and Traumatic Brain Injury Among Servicemembers | Offers a comprehensive examination of two critical and often interconnected conditions affecting military personnel.

The Art and Science of Hyperbaric Medicine | A modern, in-depth textbook that blends clinical expertise with scientific research to explore the full scope of hyperbaric oxygen therapy (HBOT).

Hyperbaric & Undersea Medicine | A specialized reference that explores the physiological, clinical, and operational aspects of hyperbaric oxygen therapy and diving medicine.

These notable books on hyperbaric medicine, span foundational texts, clinical guides, and emerging applications.

Charles Wesley Shilling was a pioneering figure in undersea and hyperbaric medicine.

Simon Mitchell is a renowned diving and hyperbaric medicine specialist from New Zealand who is internationally recognized for his research and expertise in diving physiology, decompression illness, and underwater safety.

Dr. Shai Efrati is a globally recognized leader in hyperbaric medicine and neuroscience.

The Oxygen Revolution, Third Edition by Dr. Paul G. Harch and Virginia Mc-Cullough | A comprehensive guide to Hyperbaric Oxygen Therapy (HBOT)

Doc, I Want My Brain Back by Dan Greathouse | After suffering a brain injury during a scuba diving accident in 1991, Dan Greathouse was misdiagnosed by over 30 medical professionals and then discovered HBOT.

A Lifetime at War: Life After Being Severely Wounded in Combat, Never Ending Dung by Gordon L. Ewell | A powerful memoir that chronicles the battle faced by wounded veterans long after the battlefield.

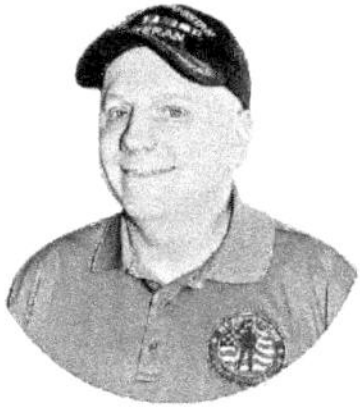

About the Author

Kevin Hensley is a retired U.S. Air Force veteran from Michigan who has become a leading advocate for veterans suffering from toxic exposure, particularly from burn pits used during military operations. He enlisted in 1995 as a Security Forces Airman and served for 20 years, deploying to Iraq, Afghanistan, Kuwait, Saudi Arabia, Oman, Jordan, and Pakistan.

After retiring in 2015, he returned to Wayne County, Michigan. During his service, Hensley was exposed to burn pits, which led to severe respiratory issues and a diagnosis of constrictive bronchiolitis—a terminal lung condition. After years of misdiagnoses, he found relief through Hyperbaric Oxygen Therapy (HBOT), which significantly improved his quality of life.

Today, Hensley serves as Co-Chair of the HBOT Committee for the Grunt Style Foundation and is a member of the National Legislative Committee for the Veterans of Foreign Wars (VFW) in Michigan. He also leads advocacy efforts for BurnPits360MI and played a key role in the passage of the PACT Act. His work includes co-authoring a book titled The Promise, and his journey continues to inspire policy change and support for veterans nationwide.

To Contact the Author...

Why Not HBOT?

(Facebook page)

www.ingramcontent.com/pod-product-compliance
Lightning Source LLC
LaVergne TN
LVHW022034200926
848481LV00007B/2675
* 9 7 9 8 3 4 9 5 8 4 2 7 5 *